I0473490

THROUGH THE EYES OF A SURVIVOR –
STROKE

THROUGH THE EYES OF A SURVIVOR –
STROKE

Brian Maram

Copyright

THROUGH THE EYES OF A SURVIVOR - STROKE

Copyright © 2022 Brian Maram

First edition 2022

All rights reserved. No part of this book may be reproduced or transmitted in any form or by any means, electronic or mechanical, including photocopying, recording or any information storage or retrieval system without permission from the copyright holder.

The author has made every effort to trace and acknowledge sources/resources/individuals. In the event that any images/information have been incorrectly attributed or credited, the Author will be pleased to rectify these omissions at the earliest opportunity

ISBN 978-0-6398387-6-2

Self-Published by: Brian Maram

Website: www.neuvare.com

Cover designed by: Brian Maram

E-mail: info@neuvare.com

Dedication

"To my loving children Thank you for your support and patience, I would never have achieved my dream without your support."

Disclaimer

This book is a work of non-fiction and is intended to provide accurate information in regards to the subject matter covered. The content is based on factual information provided to and by the author, and any similarities to other individuals, real, fictional, dead or alive are purely coincidental.

This book is not intended to be used, nor should it be used, to diagnose or treat any medical condition. For diagnosis or treatment of any medical problem, consult your own physician. The editor, publisher and author are not responsible for any specific health or allergy needs that may require medical supervision and are not liable for any damages or negative consequences from any treatment, action, application or preparation, to any person reading or following the information in this book. Neither is this book intended as a substitute for the medical advice of physicians. The reader should regularly consult a physician in matters relating to his/her/their health and particularly with respect to any symptoms that may require diagnosis or medical attention.

This book is designed based on the author's personal experience and is meant to provide information and motivation to its readers. It is sold with the understanding that the publisher and author are not engaged to render any type of medical, psychological, legal, or any other kind of professional advice. The content is the sole expression and opinion of its author and publisher. Neither the editor, publisher nor the author shall be liable for any physical, psychological, emotional, financial, or commercial damages, including, but not limited to, special, incidental, consequential or other damages. Our views and rights are the same: You are responsible for your own choices, actions, and results.

The author and publisher do not assume and hereby disclaim any liability to any party for any loss, damage or disruption caused by information, errors or omissions, whether such information, errors or omissions result from negligence, accident or any other cause.

Table Of Contents

Preface

If you are reading this book, you have either survived a life-changing stroke or you know someone who has.

Inevitably, the family will be overjoyed that their loved one survived such a horrendous ordeal. Little do they realise how unprepared they are for the complex flood of emotions the survivor is about to undergo.

Surviving a stroke is the easy part, but the life-changing ordeal that is about to follow will ultimately put the entire family through one of hell's more definitive tests. As you embark on this new unpredictable journey, the life you once knew is about to end, and the one that lies ahead of you is a life you could never have imagined. With no instruction manuals to guide you through this treacherous journey, you will find yourself having to wing it as you go.

The author, a stroke survivor himself, survived a deadly haemorrhage in the pons area of his brainstem. From that dreadful moment, the lives of his close-knit family were changed forever. No one was prepared for the mystifying flood of emotions that were about to be set into motion.

At the time of a stroke, sections of the brain are deprived of life saving oxygen, causing brain cells to die. Changes in behaviour are a reflection of such trauma. The most troublesome behaviour you will encounter is their sudden change in personality.

Acknowledgement

"I would like to thank my children and therapists without whose dedicated help and support this book would never have been completed."

CHAPTER ONE

Hospitalisation

Neurological Insults

Neurological Insults are not restricted to stroke and come in many forms. Recovering from a brain injury is more of a marathon than a sprint. Each brain injury is a unique journey that requires dedication, perseverance and patience. No two injuries are the same, and each is different and beyond compare.

Early intervention can have an enormous impact on their recovery.

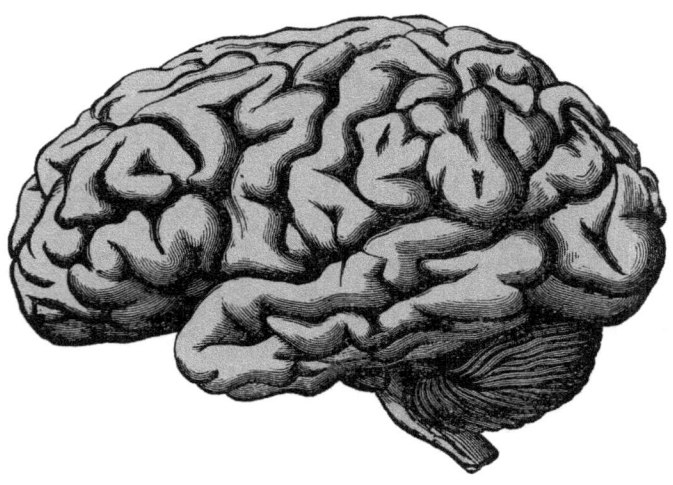

MRI

Magnetic Resonance Imaging(MRI) is a medical imaging technique used in radiology to form pictures of the body's anatomy and physiological processes.

An MRI can detect various brain conditions, *especially following head trauma.* Conditions such as bleeding, swelling, inflammation or problems with the blood vessels. An MRI can also detect cysts, tumours, developmental and structural abnormalities and infections in patients.

The MRI scanner is a large cylindrical tube that contains powerful magnets, and patients are passed through the inside of the tube during the scan.

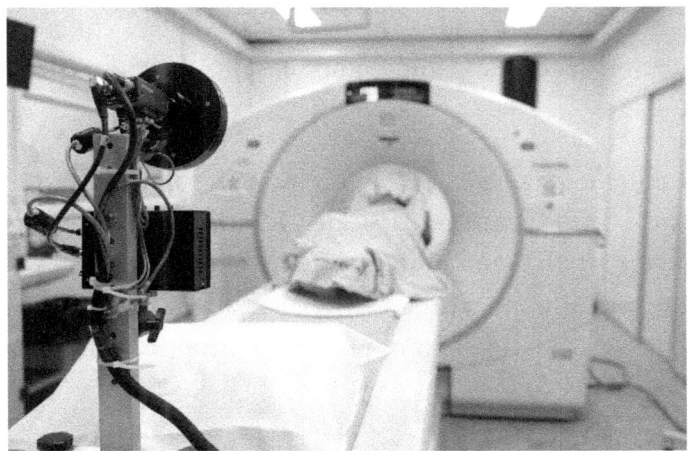

They help doctors identify what is causing a patient's health issue to diagnose them accurately and prescribe a treatment plan. Depending on a patient's symptoms, an

MRI can be used to scan a specific portion of the body for diagnosing; for example, only the brain in the case of a TBI or Stroke patient. An MRI can also help doctors to identify structural lesions.

Computerised Tomography (CT)

A **Computerised Tomography (CT)** scan combines a series of X-ray images taken from various angles and uses computer processing to create cross-sectional images (slices) of bones, blood vessels and soft tissues inside a patient's body. They reveal internal injuries and bleeding, such as those caused by a stroke. The images from a CT scan are more detailed than standard X-rays. The scans are painless, fast and easy.

X-rays, MRIs, and CT scans can detect fractures, haemorrhages, swelling, and certain kinds of tissue damage.

A patient suspected of having a stroke can have a CT scan. A **CT scan can usually identify whether they have had an ischaemic or haemorrhagic stroke**. CT's are generally quicker than MRI scans, which means that doctors are able to provide the appropriate treatment sooner.

The radiation exposure is small with one head scan. However, repeated exposure to scans over a long period can increase the patient's cancer risk. Today's CT scan technology is faster than it used to be. Therefore, the radiation exposure is less than what it once was.

That First Hospital Visit

Visiting a loved one in the hospital for the first time can be a traumatic experience. It can be overwhelming to see your loved one helplessly lying in bed, entangled in a web of pipes and cables, hanging onto life.

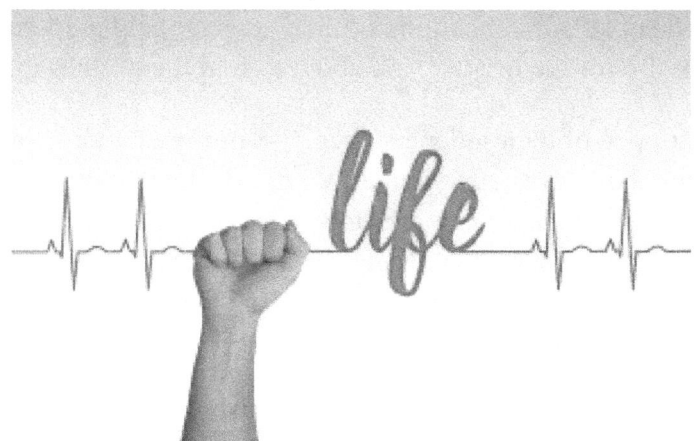

The patient may be in a coma and unresponsive. Making the uncertainty of what the future holds daunting. Everything will be in the air until such time that they awake, and only then can the true extent of the damage be accessed.

Once a stroke has revealed its ugly head. The lives of the survivor and their family are thrown into turmoil. The devastation unleashed onto them can be overwhelming and surprisingly fast. Life changes instantaneously, and the injury can come at an immense cost, not only financially but also to their health, independence and relationships.

Not many people realise the extended impact a stroke can have on the family; overnight, a partner becomes a caregiver and/or a breadwinner becomes unemployed. The life they once knew abruptly comes to a screeching halt. In a flash of light, their lives are changed forever and forever is a long time to try and envisage.

No books or publications could ever genuinely prepare a family for the life they are about to find themselves in.

Stripped of their independence, the aftermath of a stroke can be devastating and is approached with fear. Apprehension and uncertainty taint the future of those close to the survivor. With no idea of what lies ahead of them, families fear the worst knowing that they are about to be exposed to uncharted waters.

Most are unaware of the tsunami of emotions that are about to be unleashed onto them and will be unfamiliar with what to look out for. Not knowing how to handle the situation on their own, they will need assistance from a **neuro-psychologist.**

Stabilisation

The priority of the hospital following a stroke is to stabilise the survivor. Once a hospitalised survivor is medically stable, the hospital can move them to inpatient rehabilitation.

Inpatient rehabilitation may also be referred to as acute rehabilitation.

Patients who cannot meet the requirements of inpatient rehabilitation may be discharged to a skilled nursing facility.

Skilled Nursing Facility

The difference between a nursing home and a skilled nursing facility is whether they offer medical care or not.

People who require high levels of assistance with everyday living tasks and **non-medical care** would go to a nursing home. Those with acute conditions requiring **medical care**, such as stroke survivors, would be sent to a skilled nursing facility.

A **skilled nursing facility (SNF) is** a place for the elderly or disabled who require medical care and cannot look after themselves.

Nursing facilities go by many different names depending on their levels of care. They may be referred to as nursing homes, skilled nursing facilities, long-term care facilities, old age homes, assisted living facilities, care homes, rest homes, convalescent homes or convalescent care. The titles differ slightly to indicate the levels of care they offer and whether the institution is public or private.

They also indicate whether they provide mainly assisted living, nursing care or nursing care with emergency medical care.

Skilled Nursing facilities provide a solution to patients who do not need to be in a hospital but cannot be cared for at home.

At nursing facilities, nurses are responsible for caring of a patient's medical needs. Depending on their ranks and seniority, the nurses' responsibilities may extend to them being in charge of other employees. Skilled nursing facilities have nursing aides and experienced nurses on hand 24/7.

CHAPTER TWO

Brain Anatomy

Brain Structure

The brain is a complex organ and is divided into three principal areas, consisting of the Cerebrum, Cerebellum and Brainstem.

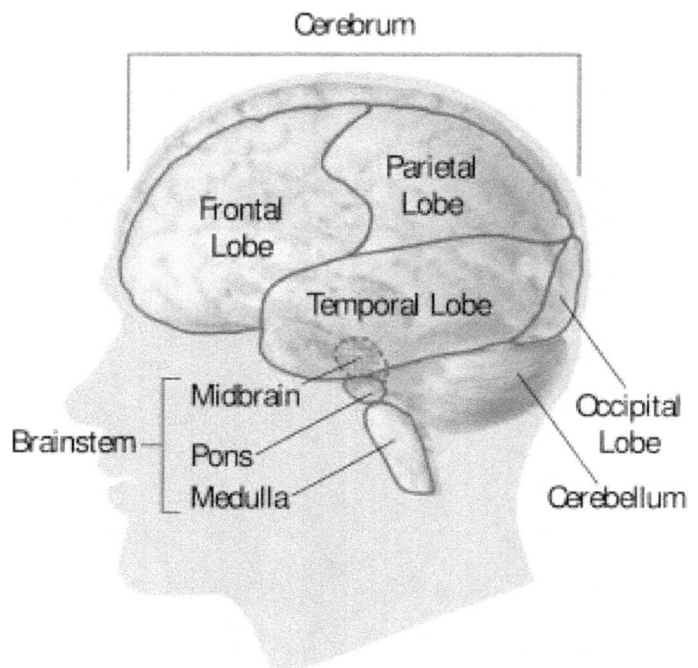

The largest part of the human brain is the Cerebrum which is divided into two hemispheres and is associated with higher brain function. Each hemisphere is made up of four lobes consisting of the Frontal, Temporal, Parietal and Occipital Lobes.

These four lobes are then further subdivided into substructures that are associated with specific functions and these have been detailed below under each description.

The Cerebellum is located at the brain's posterior and is positioned under the cerebrum hemispheres.

The brainstem is situated deep inside the brain and is a continuance of the spinal cord. The Pons, Medulla Oblongata and Midbrain make up the brainstem.

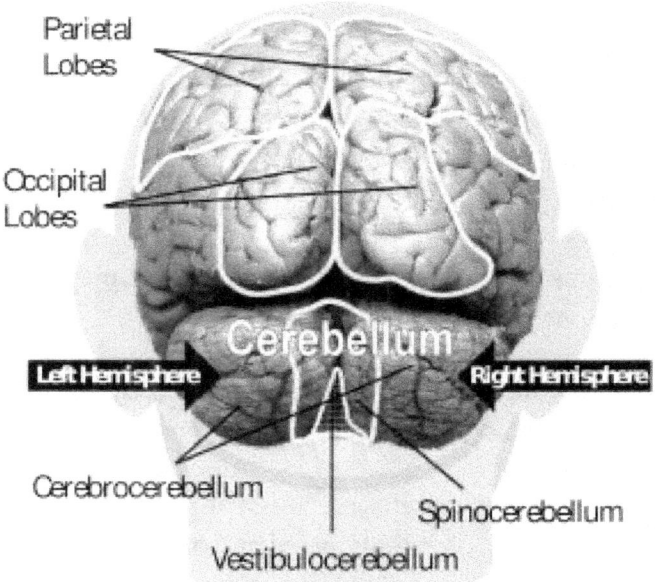

The **left hemisphere** of the brain controls the right side of the body and is responsible for **speech, comprehension, arithmetic, and writing**.

The right hemisphere controls the left side of the body and is responsible for creativity, spatial ability, artistic, and musical skills.

Frontal Lobe

The Frontal Lobes can be found in the front of the brain and makes up the largest portion of the brain. Forming part of the cerebral cortex, it is the main site for higher cognitive functioning.

The substructures that make up the Frontal Lobe are the prefrontal cortex, orbitofrontal cortex, motor and premotor cortices, Broca's area, frontal eye fields, middle and inferior frontal gyru.

Functions associated with the Frontal Lobe play a major part in one's voluntary movement.

Activities such as walking are controlled by the Frontal Lobe as it houses the primary motor cortex.

Other functions include: executive procedures (decision-making skills, planning, problem-solving, judgement, inhibition and thinking), attention and thought, voluntary behaviour, cognition, intelligence, language processing and comprehension, plus many more.

Damage to the Frontal Lobe might cause paralysis, mood changes and nonconforming social and personality behaviours. Emotions that are felt by the survivor, may not necessarily be expressed in their face or voice. On the contrary, they may exhibit excessive displays of emotions.

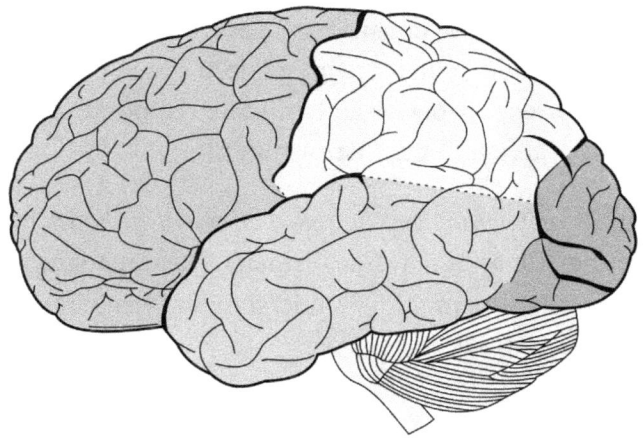

Parietal Lobe

The substructures making up the Parietal Lobe are the somatosensory cortex, inferior and superior parietal lobules and the praecuneus.

Functions associated with the Parietal Lobe include perception and integration of somatosensory information (touch, pressure, pain and temperature), visuospatial processing, spatial attention and mapping, as well as number representation.

Damage to the Parietal Lobe could cause the inability to locate and recognise objects, hemispatial neglect (the lack of attention to and awareness of one side of the field of vision), disorientation and lack of coordination.

Temporal Lobe

The Temporal Lobe consists of several substructures. These include the amygdala, the primary auditory cortex, superior and middle temporal gyrus, Wernicke's area and the fusiform gyrus.

Functions associated with the Temporal Lobe include perception (hearing, vision, smell), face recognition, learning and memory, understanding language and emotional reactions.

Damage to the Temporal Lobe may result in difficulties in understanding speech (Wernicke's Aphasia), recognition of faces and objects, the inability to attend to sensory input, persistent talking, memory loss (short and long term), an increase or decrease in sexual behaviour, aggression and difficulty recalling visual stimuli.

Dysfunction of the Temporal Lobe is closely aligned with the neuropathological disorder, Schizophrenia.

Occipital Lobe

The two Occipital Lobes are the smallest of the four paired lobes in the cerebral cortex. The primary visual area of the brain is located in the Occipital cortex. Because it's the primary visual centre, it contains most of the anatomical region of the visual cortex and its substructures consist of the cuneus and visual areas V1 – V5.

The Occipital Lobe is associated with vision and d*amage* to this area could result in hallucinations, blindness and the inability to see colour or motion.

Cerebellum

The Cerebellum is the region of the brain that coordinates and regulates motor behaviour, particularly automatic movements. It is located at the bottom of the brain and is tucked in under the cerebral hemispheres.

Functions associated with the Cerebellum include voluntary movement, motor learning, reflex, balance memory, posture, timing and sequence learning.

Damage to this area of the brain could result in the loss of coordination, tremors, inability to walk, dizziness (vertigo) or slurred speech.

Brainstem

The Brainstem is situated in the posterior part of the brain and is a continuation of the spinal cord. It is made up of structures that lie deep within the brain and consists of the pons, medulla oblongata and midbrain.

It plays a vital role in maintaining and controlling automated functions such as breathing, blood pressure and heart rate. It further regulates the central nervous system and is crucial in maintaining consciousness.

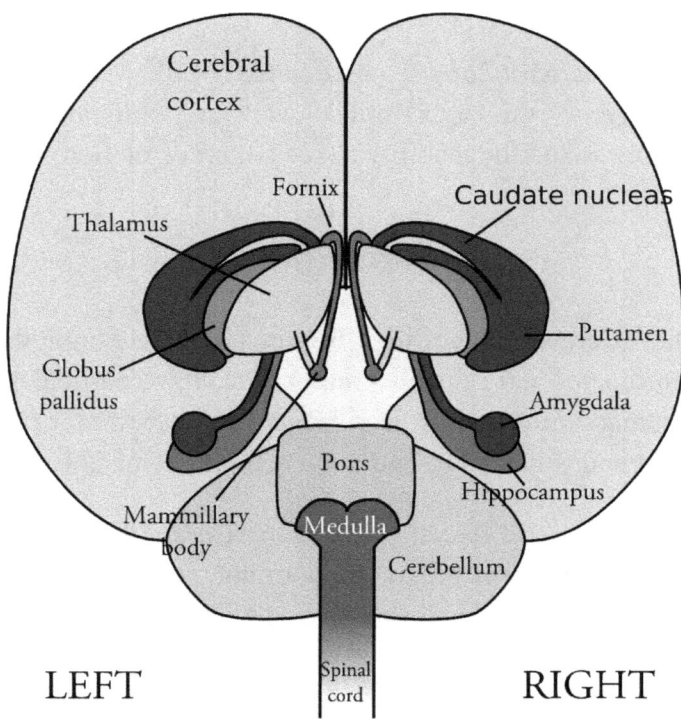

The Brainstem is *associated with* the body's automated functions (blood pressure, breathing, heartbeat, digestion, perspiration and temperature), as well as alertness, sleep, balance and the startle response.

Damage to this area could cause organ failure, resulting in death, sleep disorders (such as insomnia or sleep apnoea), difficulties with balance and moving.

CHAPTER THREE

Understanding Stroke

Types Of Stroke

Stroke strikes with little to no warning, and finding yourself trapped in the world of a stroke survivor happens in the blink of an eye.

Typically, one of two types of stroke may occur:

Either it is from a blockage or clot known as an *ischaemic stroke*

or

it's a result of a ruptured blood vessel bleeding into the brain and is referred to as **a *haemorrhagic stroke*.**

In both cases the brain is deprived of vital oxygen, causing cells to die. Depending on the severity and damage caused, the aftermath can be overwhelming.

Ischaemic Stroke

Ischaemic Strokes are the more common of the two and account for about 87% of strokes.

Ischaemic Strokes are caused by a blockage to a blood vessel in the brain. They occur when an obstruction either blocks or narrows the artery feeding oxygenated blood to the Brain. Blockages or the narrowing of a blood vessel can be caused by a build-up of fatty deposits in the vessel, blood clots or other debris that travel through our circulatory system.

Fatty deposits can cause two types of obstruction:

Cerebral thrombosis: Which occurs when a thrombus, also known as a blood clot, develops at the fatty plaque within the blood vessel.

Cerebral embolism : Occurs when a blood clot forms elsewhere in the circulatory system. If a section of the blood clot breaks free and enters the bloodstream, it can travel up to the brain's blood vessels. It will freely travel through the brain until it reaches a blood vessel that is too small to let it pass. Resulting in a blockage, interrupting the flow of oxygenated blood in the brain.

An irregular heartbeat, known as **atrial fibrillation**, is the main cause of embolism and can cause clots to form in the heart, dislodge and travel to the brain.

Haemorrhagic Stroke

A brain aneurysm is a **bulge or ballooning** in a blood vessel in the brain. An aneurysm can cause the blood vessel to leak or rupture, resulting in bleeding into the brain. This bleeding into the brain is a haemorrhagic stroke and accounts for about 13% of strokes.

A number of factors could be the cause of a haemorrhagic stroke.

These include:

- Uncontrolled high blood pressure

- Over-treatment with blood thinners (anticoagulants)
- Bulges at weak spots in your blood vessel walls (aneurysms)
- Trauma (such as a car accident)
- Protein deposits, *called amyloid build up on the walls of the arteries in the brain* leading to weakness in the vessel wall (Cerebral amyloid angiopathy (CAA))

There are two main types of haemorrhagic stroke:

Bleeding within the brain: is known as an intracerebral haemorrhage, or intracranial haemorrhage (ICH).

Bleeding on the surface of the brain: is known as a subarachnoid haemorrhage (SAH).

Transient Ischaemic Attack (TIA)

TIA'S are also referred to as mini-strokes and are caused by clots that are transient (temporary). Unlike a full-blown stroke, TIA's are short-lived and do not kill brain cells.

The symptoms are like those of a stroke but last for less than 24 hours and do not cause permanent disabilities.

TIA's should not be ignored and need to be taken seriously, and medical attention should be sought, as they are a warning that a more significant, more severe stroke is imminent.

TISSUE PLASMINOGEN ACTIVATOR (tPA)

What is Tissue Plasminogen Activator - tPA?

tPA is a clot-dissolving medicine.

When administered quickly after the onset of *stroke* (within three hours), *tPA* helps to restore blood flow to the regions of the brain.

tPA is a clot-busting medication and is the golden standard treatment for ischemic stroke. *tPA is a blood thinner and **cannot be used for haemorrhagic strokes or head trauma**.*

How does it work?

It activates the conversion of plasminogen to plasmin, an enzyme responsible for the breakdown of clots, helping to restore blood flow to the brain.

Secondary Stroke Prevention

Secondary stroke refers to someone who has already survived a previous stroke or TIA.

The prevention of secondary strokes requires a drastic change in lifestyle and eating habits, which may also involve being placed on numerous medications to control hypertension, cholesterol, diabetes, and blood thinners.

A change in diet and regular exercise should be encouraged. Where smoking is involved, it should be discouraged and it should be quit immediately.

Stress is also known as the silent killer and should be kept to a minimum. As it is, a survivor is under enough stress trying to come to terms with their new way of life. The shock of surviving a stroke is stressful enough.

Early Warning Signs - F.A.S.T

Stroke early warning signs are easily recognisable using the acronym **F.A.S.T.** If you suspect a stroke, perform this simple assessment. If any of the following symptoms are present, seek *immediate* medical assistance, as the person could be experiencing a life-threatening stroke.

F - stands for face; look for any drooping on one side of the face?

A - stands for arms; can the person raise both arms equally and hold them there?

S - stands for speech; can they speak clearly, or are they slurring their words?

T - stands for time; if any of the above signs are present, time is of the essence. *Call the emergency services and seek immediate medical help*.

Performing the **F.A.S.T.** assessment could save someone's life.

Learn and memorise the acronym.

*F*ace. *A*rm. *S*peech. *T*ime

Can The Brain Heal Itself After A Stroke?

In times past, it was believed that what a patient had not recovered in the first year or two would be lost forever. This is untrue, and fortunately for patients, damaged brain cells are not beyond repair. With a lot of therapy, they can regenerate — this process of creating new cells is called neurogenesis.

The most visible and rapid recovery is usually during the first three to four months following the stroke, after which it slows down. Recovery however continues for the remainder of the survivor's life. As the weeks, months and years pass, it slows down even more. Eventually, these micro improvements will only be noticeable to the patient.

Can you recover from paralysis after a stroke?

While **damage to the brain cannot be reversed**— through a process known as neuroplasticity and with intensive therapy, the brain is able to rewire itself. Patients experiencing hemiplegia or hemiparesis are therefore able to regain some of the motion and movement back that they lost due to their stroke. Several rehabilitation techniques can combat post-stroke paralysis.

The New Normal

What is normal?

What might be seen as normal to one person may not be perceived as normal to another.

Define normal?

Normal is ....

Surviving a stroke with complete or incomplete paralysis is devastating to the survivor and anybody close to them. The world they formerly knew has abruptly ended and the life they once perceived as "normal" has suddenly taken on an entirely new meaning. Against all odds, the survivor has just weathered a terrifying ordeal, and the family will undoubtedly be delighted that they are still alive.

Bear in mind that the survivor may no longer be able to contend with tasks as quickly as they once did. In its wake of destruction, the stroke may have caused overwhelming, irreversible damage to the brain, with devastating consequences for the survivor, forcing them to take on a '*new normal*' type of lifestyle.

How is anyone expected to know what to anticipate without an instruction manual to follow?

For starters, the survivor needs to realise that what they had before the stroke may have disappeared forever. It is now time for them to re-evaluate their situation. Take stock of what has been exhausted and what remains. Once they know what's remaining, they would have identified the foundation to start building from. They need to focus all their attention on what remains and progressively start rehabilitating themselves from here.

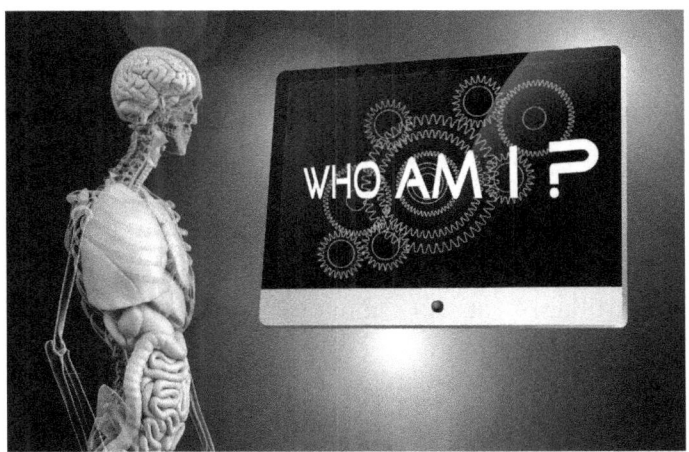

Emotional Liability

Nothing can prepare the family for the complex surge of emotions the survivor is about to undergo.

Having survived such an ordeal, they might seem like a stranger to you. Initially, the overwhelming shock of what has happened will cause them to struggle with their emotions.

Survivors are prone to intense feelings and sudden mood swings, a condition referred to as emotional liability. A survivor's emotional liability may be out of sync with their current environment and could bring on the Pseudobulbar Affect (PBA).

Pseudobulbar Affect (PBA)

The abundance of emotional liability that is building up could bring on the Pseudobulbar Affect (PBA), a medical condition characterised by the sudden and uncontrollable occurrences of laughter or crying, without any apparent motivating stimulus.

PBA is usually an inappropriate behaviour to the current situation. A survivor may find themselves laughing uncontrollably at an unhappy situation or crying uncontrollably at a joyful event.

Pain

Believe What They are Telling You

Stroke survivors can develop chronic post-stroke pain immediately following the stroke, or it may take a few months to set in.

Chronic pain can take on many forms. Nerves were damaged during the stroke, causing excruciating and continuous nerve end pain. A pain which cannot be described.

A percentage of survivors might develop Central Post Stroke Pain or CPSP, **a neuropathic pain syndrome** best described as a **throbbing or shooting pain** on the affected side. Others may experience pins and needles or numbness in areas affected by the stroke. CPSP is estimated to account for over one-third of cases of post-stroke pain.

After a while, the physical discomfort might improve so that the survivor would no longer need medical treatment.

When the author experienced this pain, the best way of describing it would be the feeling you would experience if a car door were slammed shut on your hand. However, this pain was not restricted to the hand and stretched the length of the affected side. The pain was intense and never subsided, not even for a brief period. It was with him 24/7 for many months.

Hypersensitivity

Following a stroke, the body becomes hypersensitive to stimuli such as temperature and touch.

Cold may begin to feel hot, so when something cold comes into contact with the affected side, it can cause a painful burning sensation.

On the other hand, heat may feel cool to the touch. As you can imagine, this could have devastating consequences.

Sitting on a leather or plastic-covered couch will cause you to sweat and your skin stick to the sofa. As most of us have experienced. The only difference is that when you are a survivor and you try to move off the couch, it can result in excruciating pain, giving the survivor the impression that their skin is slowly being peeled away from their body.

Be understanding of their complaints.

It is not an act, **nor** is it a cry for attention.

These painful sensations are real.

Stroke Fatigue

The biggest misconception anybody can have of a stroke survivor is that they are lazy. On the contrary**, they are anything but that.** Due of the damage to the brain, they are required to work **four times harder** to achieve what most people take for granted.

The effort invested in completing these rudimentary tasks will fatigue the most hardened survivors, compelling them to seek rest.

As a Caregiver, you need to be sympathetic to their needs by keeping this in mind. Remember what the survivor has been through and what they are currently still going through. They have no control over how rapidly they will exhaust themselves. The brain is hard at work, trying to mend the damaged paths and needs all the rest it can get.

When a survivor continually complains about the pain and fatigue they feel, believe what they are trying to tell you. Damage to the brain can bring on excruciating pain and fatigue. They are not being a hypochondriac. *The pain and fatigue are real.*

CHAPTER FOUR

Living with Stroke

Home Modifications

Modifications to the home will be necessary to accommodate the survivor's needs, whilst ensuring their safety as well.

One of the most hazardous rooms in the home is the bathroom. With its numerous sharp corners and slippery floors, grab rails will be necessary and should be fitted inside the shower and adjacent to the toilet.

A hand shower and Plastic chair are also required for the survivor to bathe safely. Clearing the area adjacent to the toilet is necessary to allow for effortless access of the wheelchair, for easy transferring.

Furniture and loose rugs should be moved around or placed in storage, once again, allowing for easy access of the wheelchair. Once the survivor begins to learn how to walk, those loose rugs and mats will become hazardous obstacles if left in place.

If you have stairs in the home, a ramp will be necessary. But before installing any permanent features, ensure that you have done your homework and that the angles are correct. After all, everything to be installed is to ensure the survivor's safety.

In the kitchen, crockery and utensils that are out of reach should be relocated for easy access. Areas may also have to be cleared, to allow for safe passage of the wheelchair.

Buffer Zone

With so much uncertainty and concern, it is natural for friends and family to call or request media updates on how the survivor is doing.

A family member or close friend should step in at this point and act as a go-between. They need to create a zone of tranquillity around the survivor.

Stress And Recovery

This chapter in the survivor's life is highly challenging, and recovery is a painstakingly slow process. Try to keep any additional stress to an ultimate minimum, as any extra pressure can only further hamper their recovery process and possibly contribute to a secondary stroke.

Informal Caregivers

The survivor might not be able to perform specific tasks that came to them naturally in the past. With a prolonged recovery process, things will usually only begin to improve once time has begun its healing process.

Your job as a Caregiver is to be there for them. Help them along this unpleasant journey by making them feel loved. Showing love and affection is vital to speeding up the recovery process.

As a Caregiver, it is your responsibility to let them know that you feel strongly about them and that taking unnecessary risks where their life and safety are concerned is not acceptable. As a caregiver, you also need to look after your health and well-being.

Evidence shows that most informal caregivers are ill-prepared for this role and provide care with little to no support—more than one-third of caregivers who continue to provide intense care land up jeopardising their own health.

Caregiving is a full-time job. It may turn out to be the hardest job you have ever undertaken, with little to no reward. Survivors have sustained a brain injury and do not always have control of their emotions. They are frustrated, not being able to do what were once simple daily tasks, but lack the control to express Emotional intelligence (otherwise known as **emotional quotient** or EQ); instead, they come over as rude and abrupt, which can be degrading at times.

Caregivers need to take time out for themselves and to spend it in a place that is their go-to zone when things get tough. They need to learn when to ask others for help, even if it's only for a few hours or a day. A burnt-out caregiver is of no use to anyone, including themselves.

Frustration Vs Aggression

The unexpected change in lifestyle can lead to numerous frustrating situations, especially with the sudden onset of a disability. To the outside world, these frustrations may be perceived as anger tantrums.

Misconstruing frustration as anger is understandable to the untrained eye. So, before retaliating and jumping to conclusions, place yourself in their shoes and try to see things from their perspective.

For example, they might be trying to accomplish something as simple as opening a coffee jar. To the abled individual, this may seem like a simple task, but to them, attempting it with only one hand can prove to be highly frustrating.

Before being judgemental, try things for yourself and see them from their point of view. Start by tying one hand behind your back and spend the remainder of the day like that. You might be surprised to find out just how difficult it is to do things with only one hand. Maybe then, you will have a better understanding as to what they are going through on a daily basis. Be proactive, learn to identify those frustrating situations before they occur.

While coming to terms with their deficits, anticipate when they cannot do something and offer to help. Even better, where possible, move things around so that they can do it themselves; after all, the best way to retrain the brain is to let them try things by themselves.

Rehabilitation is a long and tedious road. By continuously doing everything for them, they will only learn to become dependent on you and will stop trying to do things on their own.

Patience is a virtue. Reacting to their frustrations with anger will only push them over the edge, stirring up a whirlwind of unnecessary emotions. Instead, take a deep breath and remember that survivors are not in control of their actions.

Neuroplasticity

Neuro refers to the brain and **plasticity** to its pliability. Neuroplasticity is the pliability of the brain to reorganise itself throughout the life of the individual.

The survivor's family may encounter an incurious attitude from the medical staff, conservatively believing that survivors have one or two years to regain as much mobility as possible, after which there is no more hope. Such a carefree attitude and primitive belief of yesteryear are perhaps why survivors and their families give up all hope after such a short period of only two years.

The reality is that the brain, with its neuroplasticity, keeps learning over the individual's lifespan. With the brain continually trying to mend itself, recovery is possible many years after the initial trauma.

The first few months is when you will notice the most significant improvement. After that, it slows down, but it never stops.

Loneliness

Such adversity has a way of filtering out your true friends from the seasonal ones, ignorance being the principal culprit. People do not know how to act around such adversity. What are they supposed to say, and how do they react?

Human nature is to avoid such confrontations, and so they would rather go out of their way to elude any such encounters. Unfortunately, such evasions are not unique to friends. Family can also get caught up in this trap of ignorance, isolating the survivor in the process. Secluded from friends and family, the situation can rapidly spiral into loneliness and depression.

Depression

Depression is expected and easily recognisable after a stroke.

A change in mood or an aversion to activities are typical signs of depression. Survivors and their families can expect apathy from trauma to the brain. Fortunately, with modern medication, one can take pills to control depression. One should therefore not wait before seeking out medical help.

Caregivers should not take any talk of suicide lightly, and urgent professional help must be sought. The deficits brought on by the stroke may cause the survivor to become dependent on others. The sudden loss of independence can leave them feeling despondent, and they may even start to believe that the world would be a better place without them. You should not take such inconsolable thoughts lightly.

If neglected, the situation could rapidly spiral out of control. Therefore, it is of paramount importance that they talk to an experienced professional trained in dealing with such circumstances. As an independent third party, they are detached from the patient's situation; being someone who can take their hand and walk them through this taxing period.

Despite what we may expect of ourselves, we are all only human. No one expects us to be equipped to handle every curveball life throws at us on our own.

Family and friends, who have stuck around, need to reassure the survivor that they love and care for them

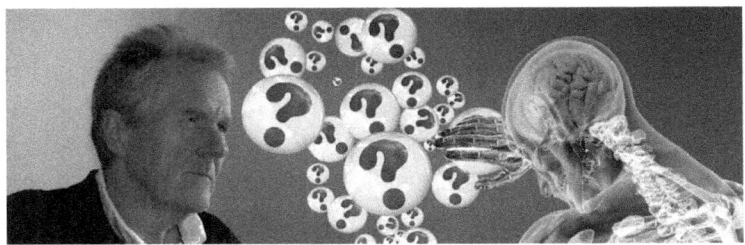

dearly. Please encourage them by letting them know that their health and safety are of utmost concern to you. It is of paramount importance that you offer as much emotional reassurance as possible.

Anxiety

After being cooped up and isolated from society for so long, while in hospital, rehab and at home. The anxiety will be overwhelming the first time the survivor returns to the community, which, incidentally, may only be a trip to the corner store. The survivor will be anxious and self-conscious about their appearance, feeling that everybody is staring at them.

Reassure them that this is not the case.

To avoid such situations, they may choose to remain

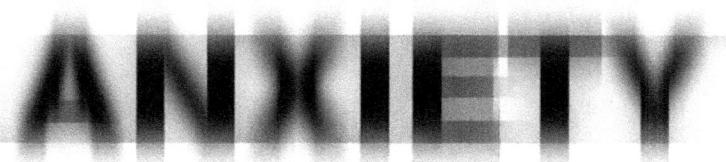

isolated in the comfort of their home.

Habitually, people are curious to find out more about what happened to a physically impaired person but are ignorant on how to approach the subject.

Rather than getting angry at their ignorance, try and educate them to better understand and let them walk away feeling wiser. Remember, survivors have been through something that they have no idea about. Instead of feeling self-conscious, hold your head up high, and be proud of who you are; you are a survivor! Not many people can lay claim to that, and no one can take that title away from you.

The good news is that the more you get out of the home, the more comfortable you will become and the less

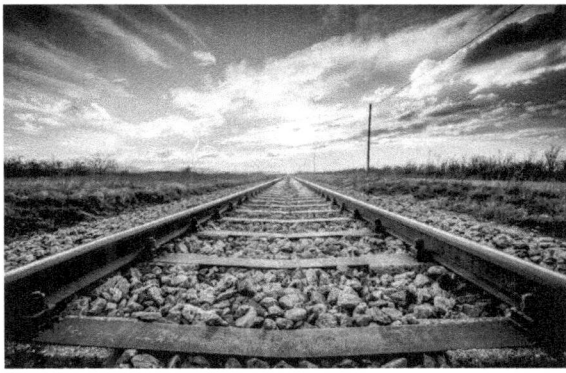

2 The way you see things

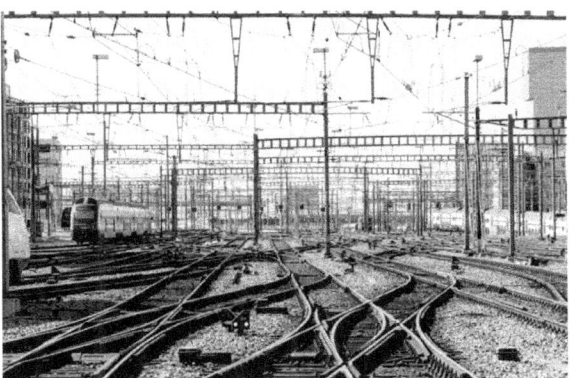

1 The way a Survivor sees things

anxious you will begin to feel. Begin with baby steps and slowly increase your exposure to crowds.

When the author initially went out into public, he anxiously paused if a crowd was approaching and waited for them to pass before moving on. The more exposure he got to the masses, the easier it got.

Exposure does heal anxiety.

Dressing And Grooming

Two of life's daily activities are to dress and groom yourself. For survivors, this basic necessity may have been taken away. Attempting these fundamental tasks with one hand can be more challenging than initially anticipated. With the aid of a caregiver, the task will be substantially simplified. Doing it on your own is another story, for another day.

Whether they have assistance or not, they need to remember to always lead with their weak side. In other words, when putting on a shirt, start by inserting the weak arm into the sleeve, followed by the stronger arm. They need to do the same with their trousers. Trying to put on trousers by themself, with a foot that will not come to the party, feels like you, the caregiver, trying to put on trousers with your shoes on.

When it comes to shoes, help will definitely, be required until, such time, they have enough strength in their leg muscles to lift the foot. In the beginning, it is easier to wear shoes with Velcro straps as tying shoelaces with one hand, although possible, is an art on its own. Over time and with some help from their therapist, the survivor will learn some tricks to achieve this. An alternative is to replace the laces with a silicon lacing system, converting their lace-up shoes to slip-on.

Grooming may prove challenging initially, especially if their dominant side was affected, but they will learn new tricks in time, and when they do so, it will get easier.

Refrain from letting them use any razors or sharp objects on their own.

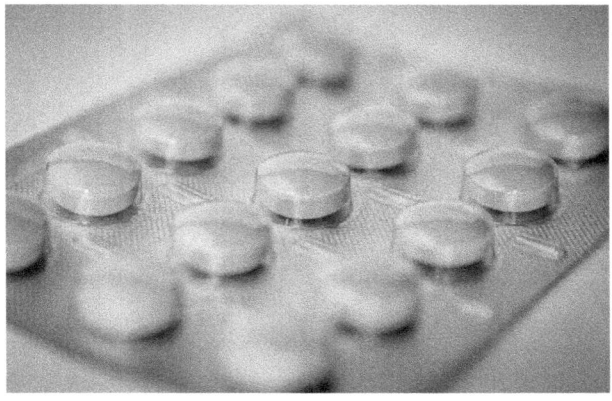

Medication And Its Side Effects

Following a stroke, the survivor may find that they have been prescribed more medications than they are used to.

These medicines come with a compilation of side effects. Sadly, these side effects can be more unpleasant than they need to be.

For some reason, it may be difficult for the survivor's family to persuade medical staff to take them as seriously as they should. Family members and caregivers alike need to **familiarise** themselves with all the medications and their intricacy.

With so many side effects, if the survivor begins to act out of character, urgently seek medical assistance and advise them on what is transpiring.

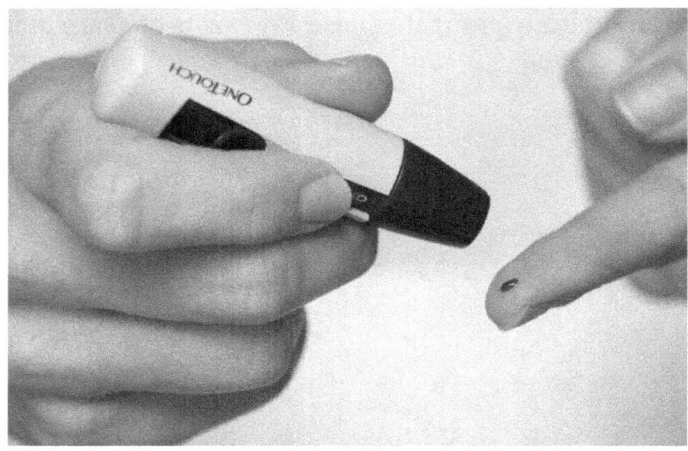

You are their advocate. *Don't let the Doctor off the hook* until they have answered all your questions and they have suggested concrete solutions.

Your only weapon is loads of questions.

Ask them,
'What can we do about…'
or
'Isn't there a different medication that…'

Intimacy After A Stroke

Sex after a stroke has always been a contentious subject and avoided at all costs. Intimacy may still be possible depending on where the stroke occurred and its severity.

BEFORE ENGAGING IN ANY INTIMACY,

PLEASE CLEAR THIS WITH YOUR DOCTOR FIRST.

Sex can be just as fulfilling as it was before the stroke. However, engaging in exotic sexual positions may prove to be more arduous, hindered by paralysis. Penetration is not everything, and with a little bit of imagination, foreplay can prove to be just as exhilarating.

Intimacy does not only mean intercourse, and you may want to start the foreplay by kissing, caressing and massaging. Start slowly, communicate your feelings to your partner, and let them know about your anxieties. With communication, together, you will be able to experiment and discover comfortable positions that will satisfy both your needs.

A Positive Mind Yields Positive Results

Don't expect everything to be okay right away.

Recovery is a deliberate process that requires arduous hours of repetition. Patience and perseverance are the keys to an effective rehabilitation.

Motivating the survivor as much as possible will get them moving, but ultimately, it's their determination to get better that will keep them going. Don't ever give up. Technology is advancing at such a rampant pace, and scientists are continually finding new ways to help survivors recover from their harrowing ordeal.

Even the toughest of the tough, the "well-adjusted" survivor who thinks they are doing well, will have some tough days. Delayed reactions are par to recovery.

Many survivors steel themselves to their loss and feel strong. That is, until the first sign of hope, be it the twitch of a finger or standing for the very first time. The slightest whisper of hope will cause a seasoned survivor's eyes to well up with tears of joy. That twitch of hope is enough to instil confidence. Hang in there for as long as it takes.

Re-enforce how proud you are of them – over and over again, session after session, year after year. Never give up hope. The more love and affection they encounter, the more determined they will recover! Recovery is a slooooooooow and tedious process; I am talking glacial speed, so don't expect overnight miracles.

Every action begins with the tiniest of twitches. The recovery process will slow down with time, but it will only stop when they, and only they, decide to give up.

Never give up, and remember that

giving up is never an option.

CHAPTER FIVE

In-patient rehabilitation

What Is In-House Rehabilitation?

In-house rehabilitation is also known as inpatient rehabilitation or acute rehabilitation.

The goal of inpatient rehabilitation is to return patients safely to their home environment. Such rehabilitation may be part of a larger hospital group or a private or government facility. Patients usually remain in these facilities for about two to three weeks.

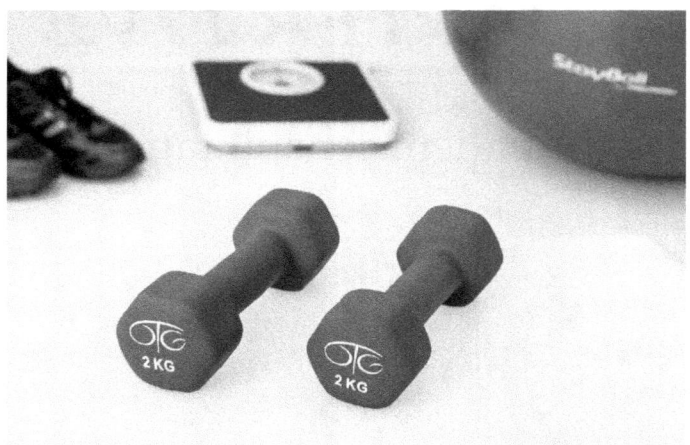

During their stay, they participate in an intensive, well-coordinated rehabilitation program. Rehabilitation is intense during this period, as the recovery process is at its peak.

In-house rehabilitation facilities are not miracle centres, and recovery does not end there. Recovering from a stroke is ongoing and can continue for the remainder of the patient's life but at a much slower pace.

It was once thought that the brain stopped healing after a year or two, but this has been proven wrong. Through a process known as neuroplasticity, the brain learns and rewires itself for the remainder of the survivors' lives.

In-house rehabilitation is intensive and consists of all the necessary therapy to hopefully get the patient home. Therapy will include Physiotherapy, Occupational therapy and Speech therapy. A Psychologist can help with the emotional side of the injury. In-house rehabilitation may also have other forms of therapy deemed necessary, such as recreational therapy, art, and music. These additional forms of therapy may also be on offer at a skilled nursing facility.

Is It Important?

The first three months following a stroke are the most important for recovery. This is the period when survivors will see the most improvement. During this time, survivors will enter and complete a two to three-week inpatient rehabilitation program, after which they will progress to an outpatient therapy facility.

On entering an in-house facility, the patient's family needs to realise that the survivor has undergone a significant change in life. The family needs to come to terms with the fact that the survivor has been taken back in time regarding their independence. They can no longer do things for themselves and need to relearn the most basic of tasks if they ever want to regain some independence.

During therapy at the in-house facility, they will be taught daily activities that most of us take for granted. Besides their daily mandatory therapy sessions, survivors will be taught how to dress and groom themselves, how to go to the bathroom on their own safely, plus much more.

In-house rehabilitation is that stepping stone to them regaining some independence.

CHAPTER SIX

Out-patient rehabilitation

What is out-patient rehabilitation?

An outpatient facility is where survivors go for continued therapy once they have completed their inpatient program. Selecting a suitable facility is of crucial importance. Therapy needs to be individualised to each survivor's needs; recovering from stroke is not a one size fits all.

Each rehabilitation program needs to be customised to the survivor's needs, and therapists need to discuss this amongst themselves and with the family.

The most successful therapy comes from a team of therapists who can get together and discuss the progress and future needs of the patient. The team needs to communicate with the family and provide regular updates on the survivor's progress.

Depending on the inpatient facility the survivor was at, they may offer an outpatient operation. A survivor could then continue with them but on an outpatient basis. If the facility does not provide this, the survivor would have to seek out an independent outpatient facility.

Searching for the correct facility may involve finding a rehab with everything under one roof or making use of individual therapists. Patients need to ensure that their therapists are *neuro* trained if going the latter route.

Is It Important?

After a brief period of intense and exhausting in-patient rehabilitation, survivors are discharged from the safe compound of the in-house facility and released back into a cruel and unforgiving society.

Formal outpatient rehabilitation is crucial at this point for survivors to regain as much independence and confidence as possible. The time and money spent on proper outpatient rehabilitation are precious, so selecting a suitable facility is critical.

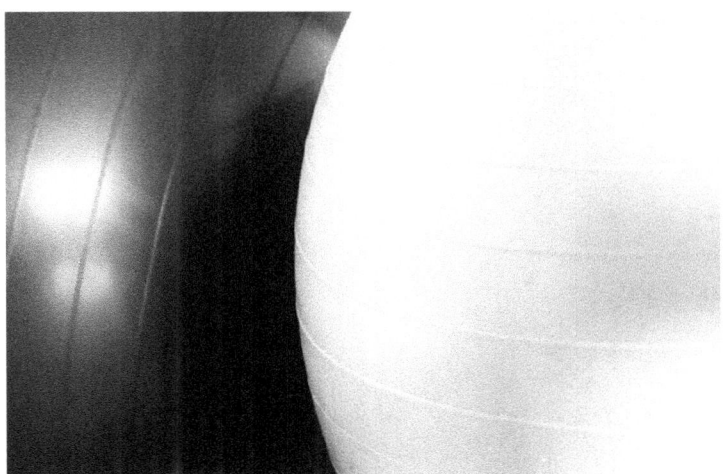

Survivors might not be able to do exactly what they did before the stroke, and rehabilitation is not a miracle cure.

Rehabilitation cannot repair damaged tissue in the brain. However, through a process known as neuroplasticity, the brain has the amazing ability to rewire itself, allowing the neurons (nerve cells) in the brain to compensate for the injury by adjusting their activities in response to the new changes in their environment.

CHAPTER SEVEN

Therapy

Physiotherapy

Physical therapy or physiotherapy (often abbreviated to PT) is a form of rehabilitation where physical intervention to an injured area is required to encourage mobility and function to re-establish quality of life.

Physiotherapists focus on the lower limbs to help survivors regain their balance and walking ability.

The lower limbs are also usually the first to respond to any therapy.

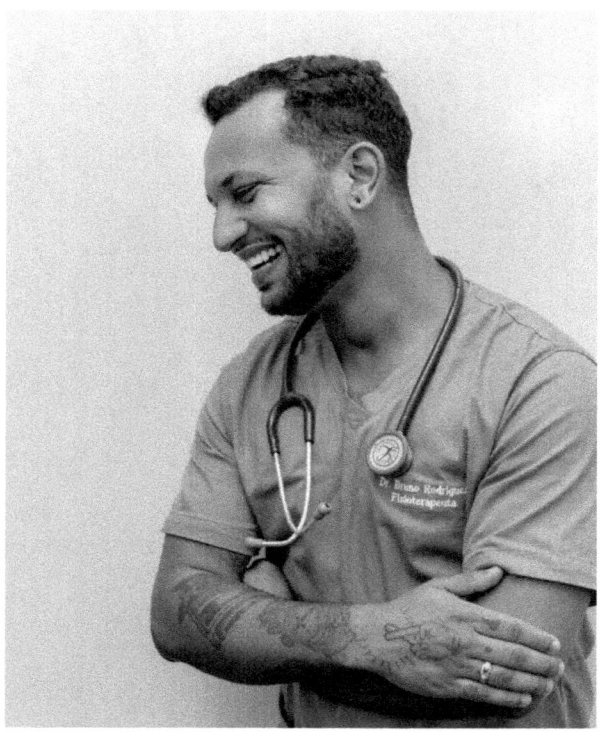

Occupational Therapy

Occupational Therapy (OT), on the other hand, focuses on the upper limb, the shoulder, arm and hand. The OT works on recovering and maintaining daily living and work activities skills.

OTs deal with people who have physical, mental or cognitive disorders. They attempt to restore a survivor's independence by identifying and eliminating environmental barriers.

They help survivors to relearn daily skills involving hand and arm movements. These skills include bathing, tying shoelaces or buttoning one's shirt.

Occupational therapists also address cognitive issues and safety in the home. They help survivors address returning-to-work issues if that is a viable option.

An occupational therapist's involvement centres on increasing participation and performance in daily activities by adapting the environment and modifying the task to teach the survivor and their family the necessary skills.

The upper limb is usually slower to respond to therapy.

Speech Therapy

Speech and vocational Therapists improve patients language skills and, where necessary, their ability to swallow. They work with patients to enhance their memory, thinking and communication imperfections.

Biokinetics

Biokinetists are exercise specialists who increase a patient's physical condition and quality of life through physical evaluations and healthy exercise habits.

Biokinetics is a step up from physiotherapy.

Both are important, and the survivor must follow the process.

There are no shortcuts to recovering from a stroke.

Psychologist

Is there a difference between a clinical psychologist and a neuropsychologist?

Yes, most definitely, a clinical psychologist focuses more on the emotional side of a patients wellbeing whereas a neuropsychologist focuses on the cognitive processes, neurobehavioral and brain disorders.

A neuropsychologist is a professional trained in evaluating disorders associated with neurological trauma.

Being detached from the situation, they are able to approach the problem with a clear mind. They are therefore able to assess whether the patients thinking skills are emotional or neurobehavioral.

Social Worker

Social workers help connect patients to financial resources and plan for their new living arrangements, if necessary.

They educate survivors and their families on entitlements, community resources, and health insurance coverage.

They are directed toward helping survivors and their families adjust to living with a disability. Where possible, they facilitate the survivor's return to the community at the highest possible functional, social and economic level.

CHAPTER EIGHT

Support groups

What Are Support Groups?

Support groups provide survivors, their families and caregivers a space to speak freely about their challenges and issues without being judged. Sharing stories with others on a similar plight can give one a sense of empowerment and control, which can reduce stress and depression. Participants may be surprised to discover just how much they have in common with each other and that they are not alone on this lonely ambivalent journey.

One of the concerns to an already tricky recovery is social isolation.

Humans by nature are social animals; who need plenty of interaction with one another to thrive. But for survivors who may have a wide range of disabilities, social contact and interaction can be challenging - even when their families are close at hand. Support groups

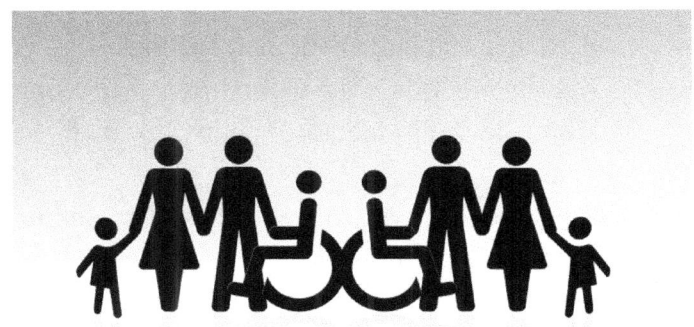

break the isolation cycle and provide a safe haven to interact with others.

Mental health professionals understand that support groups effectively cope with the stresses, changes and challenges of going through a significant life-altering event, like stroke.

Not everyone copes with neurological impairment in the same way. A support group is a great way to get to know other survivors and learn how they deal with their situation. The open, non-judgemental nature of a support group is one of the best ways to feel that they are not alone.

Benefits Of A Support Group

Support groups have numerous benefits which, include:

- They counter loneliness and isolation.
- Provide a non-judgmental, compassionate space where one can talk about their feelings.
- Give members a way to improve their coping skills and help them to adjust to their new situation.
- They are known to reduce stress, anxiety, depression, and fatigue.
- Give participants access to different information about doctors, treatments, and other resources in their community that they may not have known about.

- Help participants to make new friends who share their situation.
- Help answer questions that doctors can't.

A strong support system is the backbone of any successful rehabilitation.

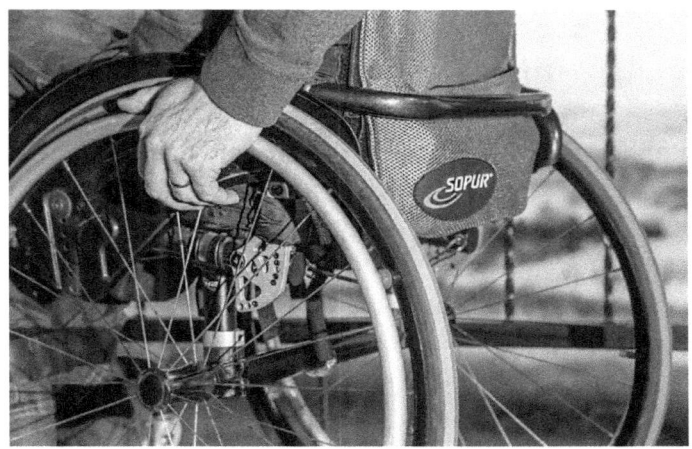

Often, survivors and their families do not know where to find assistance or whom to turn to for help. Instead of bottling things up, it is crucial that survivors have the opportunity to talk about how they feel.

Support is imperative to recovery and overcoming these barriers that prevent them from getting out and participating in the community.

They provide a comfortable environment to learn, share stories, gain encouragement and develop new friendships.

Socialising with others going through a similar adversity has proven to be a great support system.

Engaging in an active social life and relationships with friends and family is vitally important. It allows survivors to feel positive about themselves, and support groups are a perfect place to make new friends.

Are Support Groups For Caregivers

Support groups are just as important for caregivers as they are for survivors.

Caregivers can rapidly find themselves being absorbed into the life of the survivor. A support group provides a place for them to vent and helps them find an even balance between caregiving and time out.

A burnt-out caregiver is of no use to anyone.

CHAPTER NINE

Stages of grief

5 Stages Of Grief

A positive mindset is vital for a productive recovery, coupled with countless hours of repetitive therapy. Stroke is a family affliction that does not only affect the survivor. It signifies a harsh reality of the 'death' of the person you once knew and loved so dearly and the re-birth of a 'new' survivor in their place.

Learn to accept the survivor as they are. Their change in conduct could prove extremely tough and emotional for everyone. Therefore, a grieving period is required, which will lead you through various emotional stages, from denial to anger, bargaining, depression, and finally onto acceptance.

These steps do not necessarily happen in this order and can vary from person to person.

Denial

Denial is not a river in Africa; it is the beginning of the grieving process. It can leave a person feeling numb, disorientated and overwhelmed by what has just happened.

It helps people survive and get through the trauma during a stage where the world becomes meaningless and overwhelming. Life as you know it suddenly makes no sense, and you begin to wonder how you will ever continue living. In the early days following the stroke, an overpowering feeling of numbness can be expected. Some family and friends may find it hard to come to terms with what has happened and will be in disbelief. They may question how this could have happened in the first place and will carry on as though nothing had happened.

Denial is nature's way of allowing people to deal with the sorrow, and it enables them to take on as much as they can handle at a time. Questioning about what the future may hold, is a lot of hypothetical information to process. Denial is a way of slowing down this process and taking the person through it, one step at a time.

Once you come to terms with the reality of the present, you will begin to question yourself. Unknowingly you are activating the healing process and you will gradually become stronger. With time the feelings of denial will begin to subside.

Anger

Anger is a common occurrence amongst stroke survivors. Suddenly and without warning, they find themselves wallowing in a pool of uncertainty.

Stroke does not give the survivor a chance to prepare for the future. It happens in the blink of an eye and that planned future they always dreamed about, is no more.

The sudden change in lifestyle could lead to anger outbursts that may be redirected towards anybody in close proximity.

It will be towards anyone they feel they could spread the blame onto for their situation.

Their sudden loss of independence is devastating and was alarmingly fast. Trying to accept and come to terms with the deficits is just as overwhelming.

Bargaining And Negotiating

Bargaining or negotiating is when you find yourself asking many questions.

Questions such as:

'What if I had only' and wondering what you could have done differently, '

"If only I could have one more chance?"

or

"If only I had done..... differently."

Attempting to negotiate with a loss is an all too familiar scenario. Coming to terms with what has just happened is challenging.

Depression

Depression is an easily recognisable sign and is expected in stroke survivors. Regrettably, it does not only affect the survivor; instead, it touches all who are close to the survivor.

Each person will be affected to a different extent. Those not directly affected may not realise its impact on the family and what they are going through.

They might even expect them to snap out of this stage of depression and sadness and get on with their lives, which is a lot easier said than done.

The family have just 'lost' a loved one, someone they love so dearly. They need to mourn the loss and accept the new survivor who has emerged in their place. Life has just taken a drastic turn, and their future is now filled with ambiguity and uncertainty.

No one can be expected to handle such adversity on their own, and they need to seek professional help. Preferably with someone with neuro training. Someone who will understand what they are going through and to whom they can talk freely.

Seeking out professional help in light of what has happened is highly recommended for all those dear to the survivor.

A neuropsychologist is detached from the situation and trained to assist in such trying times. Having just been through a traumatic experience, there is nothing that will prepare you for the tsunami of emotional upsurges you are about to encounter.

With the road ahead being filled with so much uncertainty, you will need the assistance of someone with a clear head. Someone you can talk to, someone who can guide you through this dilemma.

Acceptance

Coming to terms with the reality of being a stroke survivor is one of the most challenging stages to acknowledge.

Admitting to a future filled with deficits and uncertainties is no easy task. Acknowledging that you might be dependent on others for basic daily living chores is no easy task.

Chores they once took for granted, that they could do with their eyes shut, may suddenly become mammoth undertakings requiring the assistance of a Caregiver. Tasks like dressing, cooking or getting around –might even require the services of a full-time caregiver and driver. Personal hygiene might necessitate the same assistance.

Try and understand what the survivor is going through. They might find themselves being powerless and resemble a child trapped in an adult's body. They may need the assistance of someone to help them bathe or wash up after having gone to the bathroom.

If you, as a Caregiver, find this humiliating, consider the humiliation that they are plagued with. They never asked to be placed in such a predicament. The stroke has put them there.

The survivor is now faced with uncertainties that they were never prepared for, be they of a physical or cognitive nature.

They might find themselves asking you many questions. Don't be intimidated by the numerous questions they might ask – no one expects you to be a medical expert and have all the answers. You are there to act as a sounding board for them, someone who will listen without prejudgement. Let them bounce their thoughts and concerns off you. Remember to always remain positive and reassure them that you will be with them, one hundred per cent of the way. Listen to their fears and emotional anxieties; after all, they have been riding a traumatic rollercoaster.

If the survivor is affected by aphasia, they might be further frustrated and annoyed by not being able to communicate. You should then speak to the medical staff about ways to communicate with your loved one.

Keep offering as much emotional reassurance as you can.

CHAPTER TEN

Hyperbaric Oxygen Therapy
(HBOT)

What Is Hyperbaric Oxygen Therapy

Before getting started, we need to understand the difference between atmospheric and Hyperbaric pressure.

Atmospheric pressure is the force exerted on a surface from a column of air above it due to the Earth's gravitational pull.

Hyperbaric pressure is an operating pressure greater than normal atmospheric pressure.

Hyperbaric Oxygen Therapy (HBOT) is the administration of oxygen under increased pressure.

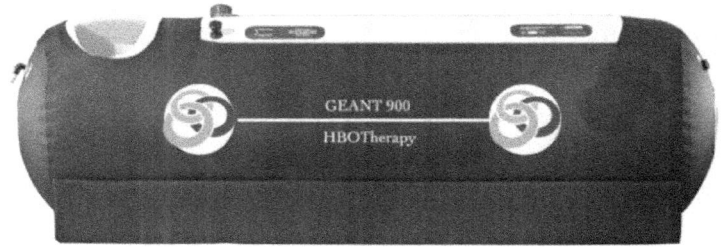

Hyperbaric Oxygen Therapy is a medical procedure whereby the body is enclosed in a full-bodied chamber and exposed to increased oxygen levels while under pressure greater than atmospheric pressure (the outside pressure).

It is a painless non-evasive procedure.

Under normal circumstances, the atmospheric pressure exerted on the body at sea level is one atmosphere (ATA).

As we ascend to altitude, the pressure begins to decrease, increasing the size of the individual gas molecules.

When we descend, the opposite happens, and the pressure increases, reducing the size of the individual gas molecules.

How Does It Work

Hyperbaric Oxygen Therapy (HBOT) works by increasing the pressure in a controlled environment (an enclosed chamber) and delivering increased amounts of oxygen to the patient.

Every day, the air we breathe comprises 21% oxygen, 78% nitrogen, and 1% inert gases. Under normal circumstances, our bodies can mend themselves using the oxygen levels found in the air. However, certain conditions require additional oxygen.

This is where HBOT comes in. During Hyperbaric Oxygen therapy, the pressure inside the chamber is gradually increased to above atmospheric pressure (outside pressure), and the breathing of pure oxygen commences. Because the body is exposed to an increased pressure, the oxygen molecules that are now also under pressure are smaller in size. Therefore, significant amounts of oxygen are dissolved into the hard-to-reach blood plasma, cerebrospinal fluid (the fluid surrounding the brain and spinal cord), lymph, bone, and other body fluids.

The smaller Oxygen molecules saturate the body and enhance the functioning of the white blood cells, which form part of the immune system that protects the body against infectious disease and foreign invaders—promoting the body's ability to aid in self-healing.

Not only do the increased oxygen levels reduce swelling and inflammation, but it also promotes the growth of new blood vessels into affected areas with reduced circulation.

Increasing the Oxygen levels in damaged tissues allows the body's natural healing mechanisms to function more effectively, even when the blood supply has been compromised.

With the aid of HBOT, damaged tissues can receive oxygen via other body fluids from surrounding areas, in addition to stimulating the release of stem cells.

Hyperbaric Oxygen Therapy is particularly effective in delivering increased oxygen to deep tissue infections with a poor blood supply.

Regular exposure to oxygen under pressure prompts and speeds up the body's natural healing process of wounds.

You may be asking why you have to use HBOT; surely an increase in oxygen would do the same thing?

You would be wrong. Remember that the individual gas molecules will decrease in size as we increase the pressure surrounding them. This includes oxygen molecules as well.

Swelling and inflammation cause blood vessels in the compromised tissue to constrict, reducing the flow of oxygenated blood to the wound.

Under pressure (HBOT), the body is able to carry those smaller oxygen molecules dissolved into the blood plasma, cerebrospinal fluid, lymph, bone, and other body fluids to the compromised tissue, increasing oxygen supply and facilitating the healing process.

HBOT Is Based On Two Partial Pressure Laws

HBOT is based on the principles of two partial pressure gas laws: Henry's **Law** and **Dalton's Law.**

Henry's Law states that "At a constant temperature, the amount of a given gas that dissolves in a given type and volume of liquid is directly proportional to the partial pressure of that gas in equilibrium with that liquid.

In other words, at a constant temperature, as the pressure increases on a liquid, the liquid will hold more gas molecules.

This theory can easily be seen in everyday use, i.e., soda drinks.

Soda effect: Soda is essentially syrup and water. Under normal conditions (one ATA), the pressure on the liquid is in equilibrium with the atmospheric pressure. By increasing the pressure in an enclosed container, we can dissolve carbon dioxide into the liquid and keep it there under pressure. Once the container has been opened, the sudden release in pressure will cause the carbon dioxide to come out of suspension in an attempt to reach equilibrium with the outside atmospheric pressure. This gives us the fizziness we all enjoy in our Sodas.

Once equilibrium has been reached, we refer to the soda as being flat.

Dalton's Law of Partial Pressure states "that in a mixture of non-reacting gases, the total pressure exerted is equal to the sum of the partial pressures of the individual gases".

In other words, the total pressure is made up of the sum of all the individual gases under pressure.

$$i.e.: P_{Total} = P_1 + P_2 + \ldots\ldots\ldots\ldots + P_n.$$

Understanding HBOT

Red blood cells are limited to the amount of oxygen that can bind with the haemoglobin (the protein in red blood cells). The plasma (the clear yellowish fluid portion of blood) only carries about 3% of the oxygen concentration.

Placing a patient into a hyperbaric environment at pressures greater than atmospheric pressure and combined with an increased oxygen partial pressure allows the body to dissolve more of the smaller oxygen molecules into its blood cells, blood plasma, cerebral-spinal fluid, bone and other body fluids.

This oxygen-enriched, saturated blood is then delivered to all of the body's cells, tissues, and fluids in higher than normal concentrations, which dramatically accelerates the healing process.

Portable hyperbaric chambers are pressurised to 1.3 ATA, being about 0.3 ATA above the outside atmospheric pressure. I say about because this will vary with altitude. 1,3 ATA is equivalent to approximately the same pressure you would experience while diving down to the bottom of a swimming pool in the deep end.

The increased oxygen concentration enhances the function of the white blood cells, boosting the immune system and promoting the body's ability to aid in self-healing.

Not only does the increased pressure and oxygen levels reduce inflammation and swelling, but it also promotes the growth of new blood vessels into the affected area.

Increasing oxygen levels into damaged tissues allows the body's natural healing mechanisms to function more effectively, even with a compromised blood supply. Damaged tissues can now receive oxygen via the blood plasma and other body fluids from surrounding areas.

Hyperbaric Oxygen Therapy is particularly effective in delivering increased amounts of oxygen to wounds with poor blood flow or injured tissue that is swollen. Daily exposure to these increased amounts of oxygen enables the body to speed up the healing process of the wound.

What Pressure Is Used?

When hyperbaric therapy was first used, higher pressures of 2-4 ATA of pressure and 100% oxygen were used.

The world of hyperbaric medicine has since realised that lower pressures (1.3 ATA as in the portable chambers approved by the FDA for use in the home and 1.3-1.5 ATA in larger hospital and clinic-based chambers) with less oxygen (often 21 to 40%) seem to have excellent effects on multiple systems of our bodies.

In particular, lower pressure appears to be more beneficial for the injured brain than higher pressure.

How long are treatments?

Treatments may also be referred to as dives and are usually 60-90 minutes per session, 5-7 times per week.

Daily treatments are required to achieve the best results.

Are there any side effects?

Hyperbaric Oxygen Therapy is a painless and non-evasive procedure with no side effects.

Some people may feel tired after a treatment. Others may experience popping in their ears. Few may have minor vision changes, but these changes are temporary.

What Will I Experience?

A patient will experience a change in pressure in their ears when the chamber begins to pressurise. Similar to that felt on an aeroplane when it begins its descent.

Usually, swallowing or yawning will alleviate any discomfort. You can also pinch your nose and gently blow. Any of these methods will equalise the pressure in your ears with the chamber's ambient pressure.

At the end of each session, the chamber pressure is reduced, returning it to the outside ambient pressure. During this stage, the ears will automatically equalise themselves.

What Is The Doughnut Effect?

Injured tissue resembles a doughnut. The hollow, middle portion of the doughnut is the traumatised area. This tissue is the area directly affected by the trauma—dead tissue in the case of a stroke. Nothing can be done to revive this dead tissue.

This dead tissue is encircled by inflamed, compromised tissue, forming a doughnut shape around the trauma, hence the name. This impaired tissue is not dead but rather inflamed, constricting the blood vessels in its path restricting oxygen flow.

The Doughnut Effect

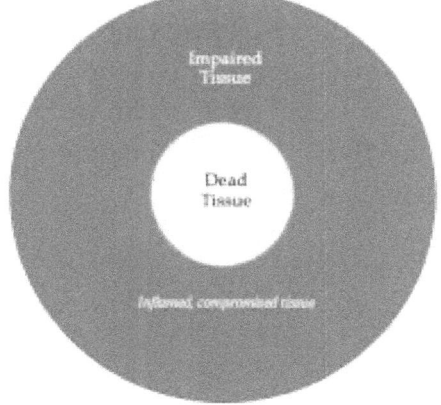

When placing a patient into a hyperbaric chamber and getting them to breathe oxygen while under pressure, it causes the oxygen molecules to reduce in size, allowing them to penetrate the compromised tissue.

The combination of the hyperbaric environment and the increased oxygen partial pressure allows the body to dissolve more oxygen into its blood cells, blood plasma, cerebral-spinal fluid, bone and other body fluids.

This increase in oxygen concentration enhances the function of the white blood cells, stimulating the immune system and *promoting* the body's ability to heal itself.

These smaller oxygen molecules can now reach the compromised tissue at increased pressures and in higher concentrations. The increased absorption promotes the growth of new blood vessels into the affected area, helping to reduce inflammation.

Increasing oxygen levels in the damaged tissue allow the body's natural healing mechanisms to function more effectively, even with a compromised blood supply. Damaged tissues can now receive oxygen via blood plasma and other body fluids from surrounding areas, initiating the healing process.

CHAPTER ELEVEN

Electrical Stimulation

Electrical Muscle Stimulation (EMS)

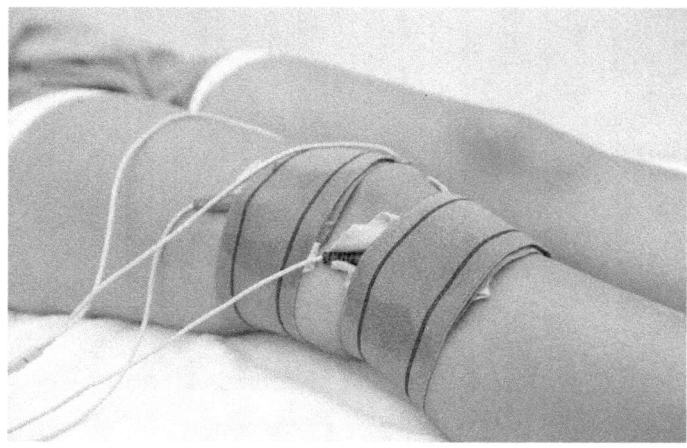

EMS uses an electrical current produced by a battery-operated device to stimulate muscle movement. The unit is connected to the skin by two or more electrodes placed strategically on the muscle. With one being positive and the other negative, the current passing between the two electrodes causes the muscles to be stimulated.

The operator can vary the intensity of the electrical current, and the device can be programmed for various cycles. Each cycle is programmed to achieve a different result.

Transcutaneous Electrical Nerve Stimulation (TENS)

TENS units also use an electrical current produced by a battery-operated device to stimulate the nerves for therapeutic purposes. TENS units cover the complete range of transcutaneously applied currents used for nerve stimulation.

TENS is used to describe the kind of pulses produced by portable stimulators to treat pain. The unit has two or more electrodes, which are strategically connected to the skin, through which a current is passed.

Functional Electrical Stimulation (FES)

Functional Electrical Stimulation is used during daily practical activities, the most common being dorsiflexion.

Dorsiflexion is the backwards movement of the front part of the foot and its digits. It is a crucial action required while walking. Dorsiflexion allows the front section of the foot to lift, allowing the foot to strike the ground on its return in the accustomed heel-to-toe action, offering stability with each step. A movement we all take for granted, and no one thinks about; it is something that happens automatically. That is, until you lose the luxury and then with every step you take, it becomes your only thought.

A traumatic brain or nerve injury could result in you losing this fundamental function, resulting in gait abnormality from the foot drop. Damage to the fibular nerve causes this. Deprived of such an essential luxury, your foot then begins to droop, and the toes drag over the ground. Providing you with the unique ability to trip over air.

When you can no longer walk in a heel-to-toe manner, the drooping foot begins to slap itself onto the ground in one movement. Besides being painful, the hanging foot causes you to become very unstable on your feet.

Foot drop is responsible for some debilitating falls. To prevent tripping, patients have had to adjust their walking gait in a desperate attempt to get mobile. They have resorted to elevating their hip and circumducting the weak leg as they walk. Circumduction is a hemiplegic gait in which the leg is stiff with no flexion at the knee and ankle. With each step, the survivor rotates the leg away from the body and then back in towards it, forming a semi-circle with each step. Such a walking gait only leads to further complications over time.

The alternative has always been to wear an ankle-foot Orthosis (AFO) to lift the flaccid foot while supporting the ankle. Not only do AFO's extend from below the knee, but they are also cumbersome and uncomfortable to wear.

Today, functional electrical stimulation (FES) units are available due to modern technology. They allow survivors to walk with a more 'natural' gait, as they help stimulate the appropriate nerves and muscles when walking.

Once programmed for your needs, the FES works with each step you take. Depending on the unit, they either have a built-in tilt sensor or a heel switch that triggers the unit every time you step on it, sending an electrical pulse to activate the nerves. Having stimulated the peroneal nerve, the front of the foot lifts and tilts backwards, allowing the survivor to walk with a more natural gait

CHAPTER TWELVE

Terminology

Easy Reference

Adult Diaper - A diaper made to be worn by adults

Ankle Foot Orthosis (AFO) - A brace used to support the foot and ankle

Anxiety - Nervous behaviour; a state of uneasiness

Aqua Therapy - Exercises performed in water

Atrial Fibrillation - An irregular heartbeat

Ageusia - An impaired sense of taste

Agnosia - The inability to recognise an object by touch alone

Agraphia - Struggle in writing or drawing

Alexia - Inability to read

Amnesia - Loss of memory

Aneurysm - The swelling of a blood vessel that may rupture and bleed, causing a stroke

Angioplasty - A procedure to improve blood flow by stretching narrowed coronary artery

Aphagia - The inability to swallow

Aphasia - A partial or total loss of the ability to articulate ideas or comprehend spoken or written language, resulting from damage to the brain caused by the stroke

Apathy - A lack of feeling, emotion and interest

Apraxia - Struggle to coordinate movement or speech

Ataxia - Loss of muscle function

Atheroma - A build-up of fatty deposits in blood vessels that restrict blood flow

Atherosclerosis - A build-up of cholesterol, fats and other substances in and on the artery walls

Arteriovenous Malformation (AVM) - An abnormal structure of arteries and veins within the brain that runs the risk of a haemorrhage

Atrial Fibrillation (AFib) - An irregular, often rapid heart rate that usually causes poor blood flow

Blood Pressure - Pressure of blood inside the arteries

Blood thinners - Medication used to thin blood

Botox - A neurotoxic protein used to ease high tone temporarily

Brain attack - A new term for a stroke

Brainstem - Posterior part of the brain and is a continuation of the spinal cord, responsible for basic life functions

Caregiver - An individual who helps another with an impairment with their Activities of Daily Living (ADL)

Carotid Arteries - Blood vessels that supply oxygenated blood to the brain and neck

Carotid Doppler - Ultrasound of the arteries in the neck to check for blockages

Carotid Endarterectomy - A procedure to clear a blockage from a Carotid Artery

CAT Scan - Computerised Axial Tomography Scan, a two-dimensional scan used to look at sections of the body in detail

Central Stroke Pain (Central Pain Syndrome) - A mixture of sensational pain that occurs after a stroke due to damage in the thalamus area of the brain. These sensations include burning brought on by hot and cold.

Cerebrospinal fluid (CSF) - A clear, colourless that surrounds the brain and spinal cord.

Cerebrovascular Disease - A group of conditions that affect blood flow and the blood vessels in the brain

Cerebral Haemorrhage - Medical term for a bleed in the brain

Cholesterol - Fatty deposits in the arteries

Clonus - A series of involuntary rhythmic muscle contractions and relaxations

Cognitive Impairment - When a person has difficulty remembering, learning, concentrating or making decisions that affect their everyday life.

Contracture - When a joint becomes fixed in one position

Cerebrovascular Accident (CVA) - The medical term for a stroke

Deep Vein Thrombosis (DVT) - A blood clot that forms in a vein deep in the body

Depression - A low mood disorder, depressed mood

Diabetes - The build-up of glucose(sugar) in one's blood caused by the inability of the pancreas to produce enough insulin (a hormone that allows the body to absorb sugar).

Diplopia - Double vision

Dorsiflexion - The flexion or extension of the foot at the ankle. The raising of the foot where the toes are brought closer to the shin

Dysarthria - Weakness of the muscle used in speaking, making communication difficult

Dysphagia - Difficulty swallowing

Dyslexia - Difficulty reading

Dysphasia - Difficulty using and understanding language

Dysphonia - Difficulty speaking at a desired volume

Dyspraxia - Difficulty coordinating movement or speech

Eccentric Exercises - In *eccentric contraction*, the tension generated is insufficient to overcome the external load on the muscle, and the muscle fibres lengthen as they contract.

Rather than working to pull a joint in the direction of the muscle contraction, the muscle acts to decelerate the joint at the end of a movement or otherwise control the repositioning of a load.

Edema - Swelling caused by excess fluid being trapped in body tissues

Electrical Stimulation - Electrical impulses are used to stimulate muscles and contract muscles

Embolism - The lodging of an embolus, a blockage-causing piece of material, inside a blood vessel

Embolic Stroke - Occurs when a blood clot that forms elsewhere in the body breaks loose and travels to the brain.

Embolus - A clot, plaque, or other material travels through the bloodstream and creates blockages.

Emotional liability - Prone to strong feelings and sudden mood swings

EMS - Electrical Muscle Stimulation

Endothelial wall - A single layer of cells that line the inside of a blood vessel.

Feeding Tube - A medical device used to feed nutrient supplements to survivors who cannot swallow. Nutrients are supplied directly to the survivors' stomachs.

Foot drop - Is the dropping of the forefoot due to weakness of the muscle

Gait - The pattern of movement of the limbs while moving, walking

HBOT - Hyperbaric Oxygen Therapy

Hemianopia - Blindness in half the visual field in both eyes

Hemiparesis - Weakness or partial paralysis on one side of the body

Hemiplegia - Complete paralysis on one side of the body

Haemorrhage - Bleeding from a ruptured blood vessel

Haemorrhagic Stroke - Bleeding onto the brain from a ruptured blood vessel, restricting oxygenated blood flow

Haematoma - A blood clot

High Blood Pressure - Blood pressure that is too high inside the arteries

High-density lipoprotein (HDL) - AKA "good cholesterol". HDL helps move the "bad cholesterol" from the arteries back to the liver to break down and leave the body.

Hydrocephalus - Raised pressure within the skull

Hyperextension - A movement beyond normal limits

Hyperlipidaemia (High Cholesterol) -Too many lipids (or fat) in the blood.

Hypertension - High blood pressure

Hypotension - Low blood pressure

Hypoxia - A state of decreased oxygen delivery to a cell

Incontinence - Loss of control of the bladder or bowel

Infarct - An area of tissue damaged by the lack of oxygen and blood

Infarction - A sudden loss of blood supply to tissue - causing the tissue to die.

Intracerebral Haemorrhage (ICH) -Bleeding into the brain tissue

Ischemic Penumbra - Areas of damaged brain tissue that still has living brain cells arranged around an area of dead brain cells that are still salvageable if reperfused.

Ischaemia - Lack of blood flow to tissues within the body

Ischaemic stroke -Blockage of a blood vessel restricting the blood flow in the brain

Lacunar Syndrome (LACS) - Medical classification of a stroke in one of the brain's smaller arteries

Lacunar Infarction - Blockage of a small artery deep in the brain resulting in a small area of damaged brain tissue.

Large Vessel Disease - Abnormalities in the large brain arteries.

Low-density lipoprotein (LDL) - Also known as the "bad cholesterol".

Locked-in Syndrome (LIS) - Locked-in Syndrome is a condition where a survivor is conscious and aware of their environment but unable to move or communicate verbally due to complete paralysis of nearly every muscle in the body; nevertheless, they are still able to move their eyes and through eye movement, communicate with the outside world

Micro haemorrhage - Small chronic brain bleeds

Mirror Therapy - Used to improve motor function after a stroke by fooling the brain into thinking that the weak limb is working.

 MRI - Magnetic Resonance Imaging

Multi Infarct Dementia (MID) - Long term confusion caused by a series of small strokes

Muscle Tone - Also known as *tonus* -the continuous and passive partial contraction of the muscles or the muscles resistance to passive stretch during resting state

Low tone is experienced as "floppy, mushy, dead weight; and

High tone is experienced as "light, tight, and strong "Muscles with **high tone** are not necessarily strong, and muscles with **low tone** are not necessarily weak.

In general, **low tone** does increase flexibility and decrease strength and **high tone** does decrease flexibility and increase strength.

Muscle Tension - Muscles of the body remain semi-contracted for a period of time in the resting state.

Naso-gastric (NG) - A tube that is inserted through the nostril of a patient into the stomach to feed a Dysphagic patient

Neurologist - A physician specialising in neurology and trained to investigate or diagnose and treat neurological disorders

Neuroplasticity - Neuro *(brain)* Plasticity *(pliability)* is a term used to describe the changeability for the brain to relearn, even in adulthood

NMES - Neuromuscular Electrical Stimulation

Nystagmus - Involuntary jerking of the eyes

Occupational therapy - Is the use of assessment and treatment to develop, recover, or maintain the daily living and work skills of people with physical, mental, or cognitive disorders.

Partial Anterior Circulation Syndrome (PACS) -The medical classification of a stroke at the front of the brain which is caused by an infarct

Patent Foramen Ovale (PFO) - A hole in the heart that did not close the way it should have after birth

Paralysis - Loss of muscle function for one or more muscles

Permissive Hypertension - A strategy where blood pressure is allowed to rise for a short period of time to ensure that damaged brain tissues receive enough blood flow. Usually no more than 24 to 48 hours

Percutaneous Endoscopic Gastrostomy (PEG) - The insertion of a tube into the wall of the stomach to feed Dysphagic patients

Platelets - Colourless blood cells that help the blood to clot.

Pneumonia - An infection in one or both of the lungs.

Post Stroke Fatigue - Often confused with the misconception of being tired and lazy.

Positive Emission Tomography(PET) -A detailed scan of the brain

Physiotherapy - Is a physical medicine and rehabilitation speciality that remediates impairments and promotes mobility, function, and quality of life through examination, diagnosis, prognosis, and physical intervention

Posterior Circulation Syndrome (POCS) -The medical classification of a stroke at the back of the brain which is caused by an infarct

Pseudobulbar Affect (PBA) - Emotional liability resulting in uncontainable outbursts of laughter or crying for no reason

Psychologist - A professional trained to evaluate behavioural and mental disorders

Pulmonary Embolism (PE) - A blockage of an artery in the lungs caused by blood clots that travel from elsewhere in the body.

Repetition - The act of repeating over and over

Rehabilitation - Specialised healthcare dedicated to improving, maintaining or restoring physical strength, cognition and mobility with maximised results[6]

Seizure - A sudden uncontrollable electrical disturbance in the brain

SCD (Sickle Cell Disease) - A red blood cell disorder where a sudden defective protein causes the red blood cells to become stiff and sticky instead of flexible and form a sickle (C shape) or a crescent.

Small vessel disease - The thickening and disease of tiny arteries deep in the brain reducing the flow of oxygen-rich blood

Stenosis - Narrowing of an artery due to plaque build-up within the artery.

Stroke - occurs when there is poor blood flow to the brain. There are two types of strokes:

Haemorrhagic stroke - when a blood vessel in the brain ruptures

Ischaemic stroke- where a blood vessel is blocked, restricting blood flow

Subarachnoid Haemorrhage - A ruptured blood vessel that is bleeding into the space surrounding the brain

Spasticity - Is a feature of altered skeletal muscle performance with a combination of paralysis, increased tendon reflex activity and hypertonia; It is also commonly referred to as an unusual "tightness", stiffness, or "pull" of muscles.

Speech Therapy - Specialises in evaluating and treating communication disorders, voice disorders, and swallowing disorders.

Subluxation of the Shoulder - Partial or incomplete dislocation of the shoulder

TBI - Traumatic Brain Injury. A stroke is classified as a TBI

TENS - Transcutaneous Electrical Nerve Stimulation

Thalamus - The section of the brain that deals with sensation

Transient Ischemic Attack (TIA) - AKA a mini-stroke. Caused by a clot, they are transient (temporary), lasting less than 24 hours

Thrombolysis - A Clot-busting drug that is used to dissolve a blood clot which is causing an Ischaemic Stroke

Thrombosis - Blockage in a blood vessel due to a blood clot

Thrombus - A blood clot that forms in a vessel and remains there.

Total serum cholesterol - A combined measurement of a person's high-density lipoprotein (HDL) and low-density lipoprotein (LDL).

Total Anterior Circulation Syndrome (TACS) - The medical classification for a large stroke at the front of the brain caused by an Infarct

Vasospasm - occurs when a blood vessel narrows, blocking blood flow

Vertebral arteries - A major artery on either side of the neck that runs through the spinal column in the neck and supplies blood to the back of the brain and spine.

Vertigo - Abnormal sensation of movement, dizziness

About the Author

AUTHOR'S NAME: Brian Maram

Website: www.neuvare.com

At the age of forty-six, in the prime of his life. The author survived a life-changing, near-fatal haemorrhagic stroke to the Pons area of his Brainstem.

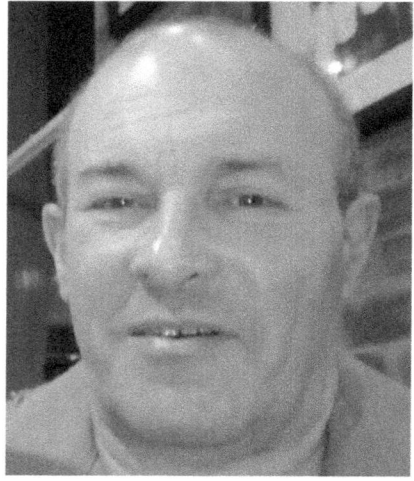

The devastation left behind in its wake of destruction was inconceivable.

At the time of his stroke in 2011 and now a young stroke survivor, there were no easy reference books to turn to for help. Brian and his family were isolated and had no one to confide in. They had never been exposed to stroke, making it all foreign to them. With nobody to consult, they were not prepared for the emotional turmoil that was to follow.

After a rollercoaster encounter, Brian found himself abandoned and alone. Isolated, he was forced to face the mammoth task of recovering alone.

Other Books By (Author)

- The stroke survivors Handbook
- Through The Eyes of a Survivor – Traumatic Brain Injury

Can I Ask A Favour?

If you enjoyed this book, found it useful or otherwise then I'd really appreciate it if you would post a short review on Amazon. I do read all the reviews personally so that I can continually write what people are wanting.

If you'd like to leave a review then please use the QR Code below to visit the link:

Thanks for your support!

www.ingramcontent.com/pod-product-compliance
Lightning Source LLC
Chambersburg PA
CBHW072212170526
45158CB00002BA/560